Protecting Your Heart While Negotiating With Your Ovaries

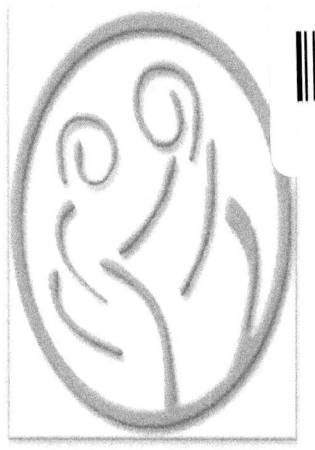

Created by:

Cristina P. Treadway

Contributions by: Gail Johnson Payne, James Payne
Treadway and Roger M. Payne

*"Working to put parenthood
within reach"*

Let's Start Negotiating

Congratulations! You have decided to be proactive in dealing with fertility challenges as you work to achieve your goal and complete your dream of having a family. This resource was designed to help you through the psychological maze associated with fertility treatment. We use the word "maze" because infertility issues can, and usually do produce many questions, thoughts and emotions that are at times, highly stressful and confusing.

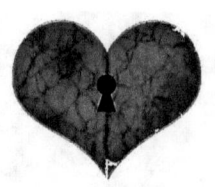

- What your personal expectations are regarding treatment and identify those of your partner?
- What you are looking for from your partner as you journey through fertility treatment?
- Answers to enhancing your relationship
- How to emotionally survive medical procedures like IUI or IVF
- How to best help your partner through the fertility treatment.
- How to deal with well-meaning friends and family.
- Learn about the mind/body connection.

- How you and your partner can deal with all possible treatment outcomes.
- Learn how to identify and respect your relationship's limits and boundaries
- How you and your partner can cope with unexpected physician recommendations while making the right treatment decisions.

Remember, there is no right or wrong answer in this interactive resource guidebook, rather, just your personal feelings. Be as honest with yourself as possible. The answers to these questions are essential to self understanding and the health of your relationship. You are already aware of the dangers to your relationship because of the unique stressors you have already faced on your infertility journey.

We challenge you to be honest with yourself and your partner as you read this book and consider the issues raised. This exercise is intended for your own personal benefit, feelings of confidence and well being in your relationship during and after the fertility treatment process. I learned a very long time ago, that "your feelings are your feelings" and they are never right or wrong, they are just your feelings. It is more important to examine the thoughts behind those feelings in order to get to the root of your beliefs.

It is in this manner that you can begin to identify your thoughts and ultimately change the maladaptive ones.

So let's begin thinking about you……

Time to focus on "Protecting Your Heart While Negotiating With Your Ovaries".

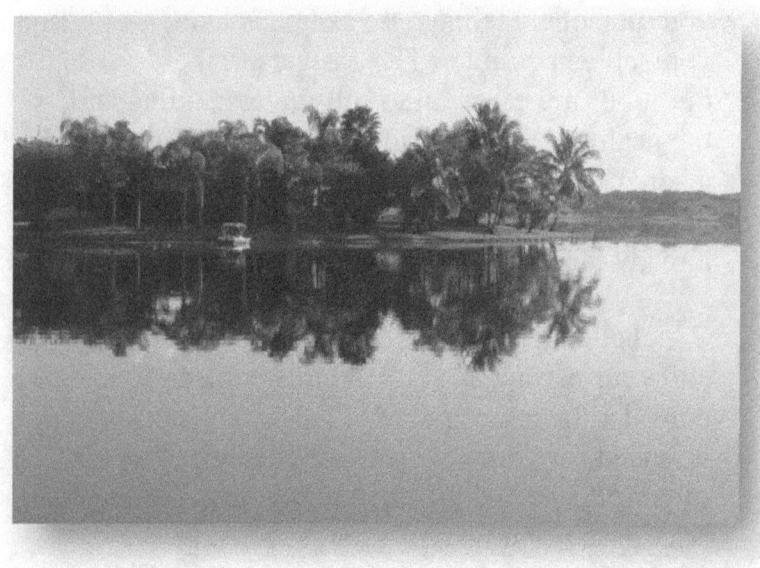

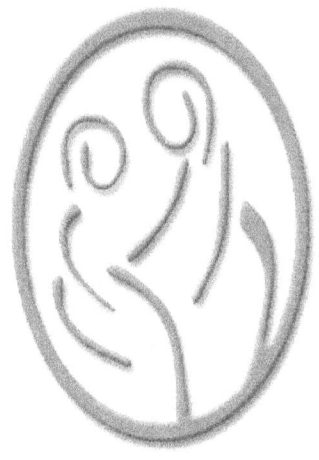

Where Did Your Ideas of Family Come From?

Before you understand the factors involved in dealing with fertility problems, you must understand your own expectations about creating a family. We are a product of our experiences and as such, our past impacts our expectations for the future. Were you a product of a small family or a large one?

- Was your childhood ideal or laden with disappointments or loss?
- Did you have a positive role model of the same gender?

_____

_____

_____

_____

_____

_____

_____

_____

Understanding from where you came will help you as you focus on where you are going and the reasons behind those goals. Understanding what ideas are behind your concept of a family will enhance your understanding of what motivates your drive for a family. Depending on those answers, you may be trying to re-create the family of your childhood memories or you may be attempting to create the family you wish you had as your family of origin.

Now consider the same questions for your partner.

- What was their family experience like, what contributed to how they think about a functional family unit?

- Was your partner's family large or small?
- Were family events like birthdays and holidays given special significance? How does this compare to your experience?
- When you think about both of your childhood experiences and your ideas about how children impact the family, can you identify the similarities and the differences?

_____

_____

_____

_____

_____

_____

_____

_____

_____

Your answers to these questions will play an important role in each of your beliefs about what family means and the importance of children in that group. Further understanding what motivates your partner as compared to what motivates your own family concept will enable you to look at the "big picture". Couples often skip this vital step as they attempt to adaptively cope with fertility problems. They know what they want, but they lack insight into the historical components that contribute to their behavioral motivation. Understanding those differences between individuals that comprise a couple, will help make the fertility journey manageable.

Infertility as a concept is a crisis that can significantly impact the health and well being of any relationship. The diagnosis and the realization that your life script and expectations are not being realized as you had planned is traumatic. It is important that you not only begin to identify your own personal feelings about the diagnosis of infertility, it is also important to try and understand what you partner is thinking about the diagnosis and what he or she perceives the health of the relationship to be. Do you know what they think and feel or do you just think that you understand?

From the days of the caveman, certain roles have been assigned to men and women respectively. Men were the hunter's and women were the nest builders and caretakers. The male initiated courtship of the female, and the woman then picked her mate from many suitors. Women chose the male who would be the best caretaker and provider. This primal dance all focused on choosing a mate who would ensure the conveyance of the individual's genes. We have progressed as a society far from the caveman days, but choosing a mate still involves the premise of passing genes to the next generation. Generally, women still have inherent desires to be caretakers and nurturers, and men aspire to provide, problem solve and protect. Of course there are differences and not all men and women fall into these roles, but they are primal forces pushing us toward creating and raising offspring.

When we have preconceived ideas of what is considered "normal" and viewed as acceptable, it is disturbing and stressful to us when we find we cannot fulfill our role as dictated by society and in our own heart. These feelings can and usually do lead to anxiety and stress. Share your feelings with your partner about your diagnosis of infertility. As a couple as well as an individual, this is a

very important step
to take as you begin
your fertility
journey.

Studies have shown
that our
personalities are
largely formed by
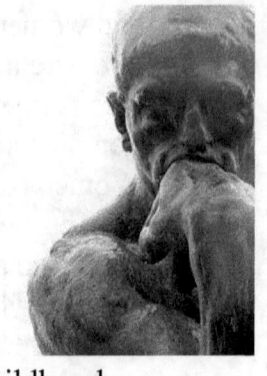
the age of five. Our childhood
experiences help influence our decision
whether to have a family of our own,
how large of a family to have, and how
we would like our family to function. It
is important to identify these feelings and
to discuss them with your partner. You
may find that your concept of the ideal
family and your partner's concept are not
necessarily the same. Understanding and
compromise are the key issues before
going forward with any medical fertility
treatment.

Of course our culture plays a role in how
we define the specific components that
are vital to creating a family. Our
culture constantly delivers messages to
young men and women about gender role
expectations. Not surprising here is that
men and women often have very
different expectations about family.

This is not to say that it is more important to one gender than the other, but rather the ways we view having a family are emotionally charged very differently. Fertility challenges may have very different thoughts behind them for each partner. Cultural messages about the importance of the maternal role verses that of the financial provider are abundant. These societal messages may seem outdated and perhaps not even politically correct; however, we must recognize they are still ingrained in our cultural foundation and personal subconscious.

Things to consider:

- Think about how important overcoming this fertility issue is to you. How important is it for your partner? How do you think this will affect you if your goals are not realized... how about your partner?
- Do you think about your fertility issues frequently, occasionally, or seldom...what about your spouse?

- What is the emotional impact or consequences of this for you? What are the emotional consequences for your spouse?

  _____
  _____
  _____
  _____
  _____
  _____
  _____
  _____

- What are your expectations for achieving your family? How did you think these expectations will manifest themselves? How far would you go to achieve your goals, are there any boundaries or limitations? Are there limitations for your partner?

It may seem obvious to ask yourself these questions, but I have routinely found in counseling sessions, that the couple I am treating has not discussed any of these questions.

In fact, they don't have a solid understanding of all of these questions as they relate to one another.

_____

_____

_____

_____

_____

_____

_____

_____

_____

_____

_____

_____

_____

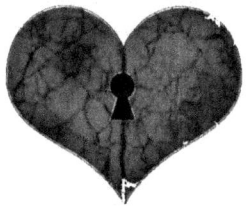

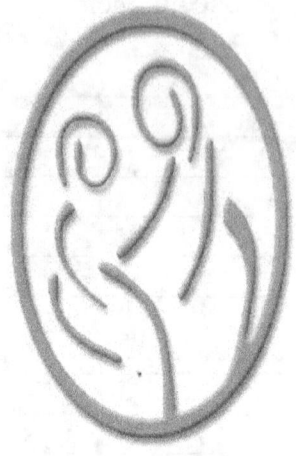

What is Infertility?

(Besides being unfair, unexpected and unforgiving)

Infertility, by definition is the inability to become pregnant and have a baby.

The American Society of Reproductive Medicine defines infertility as "a disease of the reproductive system that impairs one of the body's most basic functions: the conception of children. Conception is a complicated process that depends upon many factors: on the production of healthy sperm by the man and healthy eggs by the woman; unblocked fallopian tubes that allow the sperm to reach the egg; the sperm's ability to fertilize the egg when they meet; the ability of the fertilized egg (embryo) to become implanted in the woman's uterus; and sufficient embryo quality. Finally, for the pregnancy to continue to full term, the embryo must be healthy and the woman's hormonal environment adequate for its development. When just one of these factors is impaired, infertility can result." *http://www.asrm.org/Patients/faqs.html# Q1:*

The official definition sounds so technical. In fact, everything related to infertility sounds technical and scientific rather than natural and normal. A recent first lady of the United States asked the question and also wrote a book asking "how many people does it take to raise a child" and her answer was that" It Takes a Village". The question could then be asked, how many people does it take to create a child and a family? The answer is sometimes two, and sometimes many more than two, perhaps even a whole medical staff.

With fertility treatment it takes more than two, (but less than a village) the process can sometimes seem depersonalized and highly technical. It is vital to know the emotional temperature of your partner.

Heart Tip: Know what your partner is feeling at the onset of this journey and keep checking as the journey continues.

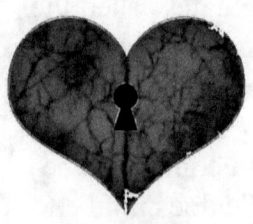

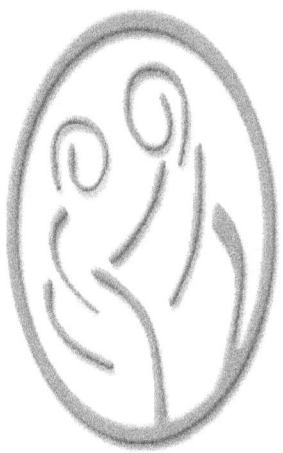

Emotional Status –Everything Can Feel Upside Down….

Infertility represents a loss of control in your life.

1. Using as many single word adjectives as you can, describe how you feel about your diagnosis of infertility?

_____

_____

_____

_____

_____

2. Looking at this list of descriptive words, can you identify any of the thoughts you have about that list?

_____

_____

_____

_____

_____

_____

_____

_____

This is not a crisis for only one partner; rather it is a crisis for you as a couple and your relationship. If you can address these challenges as a united team, the journey will be less dangerous for the well being of the relationship.

Heart Tip: If you don't deal with your emotions, they will deal with you.

How do you feel about what you are experiencing? Do you have a handle on your emotional status or are you feeling "out of control" and confused by what you are thinking and feeling? It is normal to feel like someone has pulled the proverbial rug out from under you. It is also very normal to feel like your self-concept has been negatively influenced by the infertility label and lonely diagnosis. Often the determining factor for the degree of negative impact is correlated to who has the fertility challenge. Regardless of male factor or female factor diagnosis, women often feel extreme frustration with the inability to naturally get pregnant.

_____
_____
_____
_____
_____
_____
_____
_____

Meet Rosie:
I recall a counseling session which was characteristic of so many hour sessions

with young women who were dealing with fertility challenges. I remember twenty-nine year old Rosie describing her feelings vividly, after four years of treatment.

> "I feel so stupid, I used protection for years… you know…it was dumb because I can't get pregnant, but I was so careful".

She would describe her relationship with her spouse of six years and she would reflect on her view of herself.

> "I feel broken or damaged… I don't feel attractive or desirable anymore. I have even asked my husband if he wants to divorce me, because I can't give him children. I feel like a failure as a woman, like I said, broken".

This may sound extreme, but Rosie had become depressed and very distraught due to the inability to become pregnant. She complained that her daily thoughts were largely consumed by her fertility challenge and she was unable to avoid the constant obsessive thoughts. Rose was reacting in a very normal way to the intense emotion that she was experiencing as a result of not becoming pregnant.

We would discuss all things related to infertility:
Baby showers, intrusive family, stress, frustration, inappropriate comments from well intended friends, anger, injections, medications, physicians and coping skills.

However, the one topic that always emerged as a primary concern was the effects of infertility on her relationship with her spouse Marc. This journey had impacted their intimate relationship, their friendship and tested the quality of their communication. Rosie noted the loss of privacy and the personal intrusion of the medical team into their bedroom.

> "Sex is something we do because we were instructed to do, that makes it loose something for me. Intimacy is impossible to achieve when you have your doctor's office in the bedroom with you". "I feel very alone in this… Marc is very practical and he is always looking for our plan. He doesn't understand me or what I am feeling, in fact he actually said "just relax and this will work itself out."

Her spouse was not able to grasp how she felt or why this was having such a negative effect on his wife of six years.

Rose's partner Marc ………
Marc loves Rosie very much. He is dedicated to her and would like to have a family with her. Marc describes the couple's problems with fertility in the following way:

"Rosie and I have had a really hard time with this fertility problem, she has really changed since this became part of our lives. It is important to me, but it is not everything to me. That isn't the case for my girl… this is everything to her, it has impacted every aspect of our life, that is all she seems to think and talk about. I was happy with our lives before this and I would be happy if it doesn't work out".

Men and women often experience this issue differently. Men generally approach fertility problems like they handle other life challenges… like a logical problem that needs to be solved. Women often feel fertility issues as a significant life event that is not being realized.

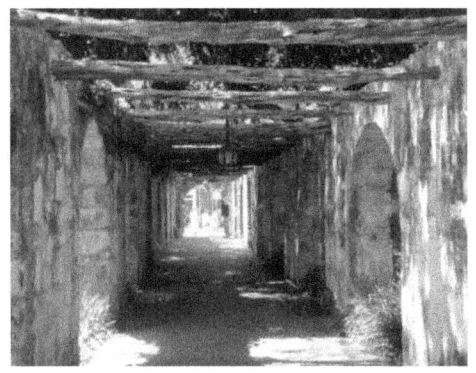

This life event is wrapped around her identity of self and what role she plays in the world. Determining to what degree individuals are experiencing this problem and an awareness of their partner's experience, will determine how effectively they can cope with the many fertility challenges. In other words, knowing how this challenge is impacting your partner and how your partner is approaching the issue will give you tools to adaptively cope.

This is an important step because making decisions about treatment options is easier when a couple is on the same page. You don't need to be at the same place on the page, but being on the same page is far better than being in different chapters of the same book.

<u>Some Exercises to Find Your Page:</u>
You and your partner each take out a separate piece of paper and answer the following questions about each other.

- How important is having a baby to your partner?
- How does your partner deal with the emotions associated with infertility?
- Does your partner feel supported by you in dealing with this issue?
- What does your partner need from you to feel supported?

You probably guessed that the next step to this exercise is to compare notes. Take turns and read your answers to each other. If an answer surprises you, discuss it objectively, without judgment. This is best accomplished by clarifying your needs but using constructive "I" statements, not accusatory "you" statements.

Remember Rosie and Marc? They did this activity in my office during a session.

Rosie was able to express what she needed from Marc to feel better supported and cope with the emotional issues associated with infertility.

Rosie: "Actually, I need you to listen to me when I talk about my feelings without you telling me how to solve the problem". "I want you to hear me and let me cry or scream…. I need you to just listen, not fix it."

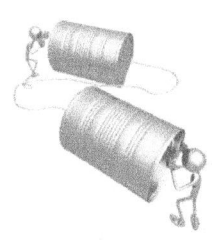

Marc: "I need to have time when our treatment and infertility isn't the only thing we discuss". "I need you to still focus on me, us and our relationship." "I feel like we are losing that magic between us that made us want a family in the first place.""I'm saying I miss us before infertility."

The exercise opened the door for Rosie and Marc to learn more about one another and how to offer the support their partner actually wanted, rather than the support they thought their partner needed. The couple was able to decide on setting special time aside to discuss treatment and all of Rosie's thoughts and feelings. They also decided on special time focused just on each other. This was scheduled time for romantic dinners, cooking together, taking a walk or going to the movies. This plan gave each of them something that was missing in their relationship. Rosie was able to make a significant breakthrough in their relationship when she realized she needed to ask for what she needed. On some level, she had expected Marc to "just know" what she needed and wanted from him, but seldom had she ever just asked.

If you can slow down and ask questions and listen to the answers, you can help each other survive. You will navigate your way down the infertility road, but the secret to how scraped up you are at the end will largely depend on how well you and your partner communicate.

Heart Tip: Slow down and listen… really listen and hear the meaning behind the words.

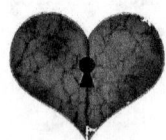

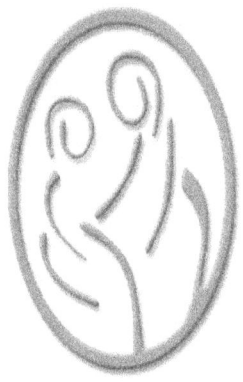

Communication

"Seek first to understand, then to be understood"

From the beginning of time, all living creatures have had some form of communication, a way of sharing wants and needs. It doesn't matter if you are from Mars or Venus, you are a "being" who communicates.

Communication is the key to surviving the psychological aspects of infertility. Remember that communication has two components. Sharing your feelings is one, but listening with compassion, respect and an open mind is the other. A mutually satisfying relationship and successful journey through fertility treatment can only be achieved with both of these components existing simultaneously.

- Do you feel that you can tell your partner your honest feelings and discuss your fears pertaining to infertility? Has your partner shared his/her feelings and fears about the infertility treatment process and outcome with you?

_____
_____
_____
_____
_____
_____
_____

- Can you identify what you need from your partner? Can you communicate what you need by simply asking? I need you to support me by...

_____

_____

_____

_____

_____

_____

_____

_____

Do you need for them to tell you what to do, how to handle things or how you should feel? Chances are that that would not be helpful. You ought to consider sharpening your active listening skills. Active listening requires truly listening to what someone says and then reflecting the message back or summarizing the message back to the communicator. This allows for clarification of misunderstanding and improved understanding.

Make a point to tell your partner exactly what you need from them related to communication. Do you need them to listen more, question more or criticize less? Do you think it would help if your partner would not offer a solution to everything you discuss?

Can you communicate how your partner can support you by learning active listening skills rather than offering logical solutions?

_____

_____

_____

_____

_____

_____

_____

Complete these statements and then communicate them to your partner.

I am feeling _____. In order to feel more supported, I need you to

_____. It would help me the most if you could

_____when I need to talk about my feelings and treatment.

_____

_____

_____

_____

_____

_____

_____

_____

Of course there is reciprocity with communication and you need to ask your partner how you can better help and support him. This may involve setting time limits for conversations or setting special time aside in the week to discuss anything infertility related.

Heart Tip: Schedule time to talk about treatment and options. Never take this time for granted.

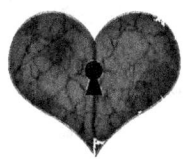

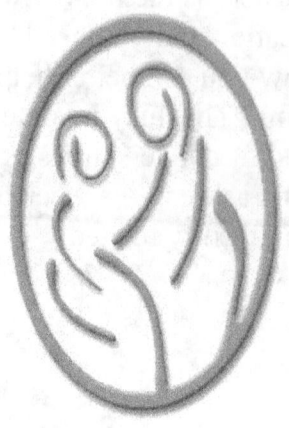

Family and Friends

Have you heard these well intentioned statements before?

- "Just relax and you will become pregnant."
- "You're trying too hard."
- "Put it out of your mind, you're thinking about it too much."
- "Go on vacation and everything will work out."
- How about this one? "Go adopt a child and you are sure to get pregnant!"
- "Your biological clock is ticking."

- "What are you waiting for, you're not getting any younger."
- "Are you sure that you are doing it right?" (This is where they want to know if you know how to make love to your partner)
- "Oh, how I would love to be a grandparent!" "When are you going to make that happen?'

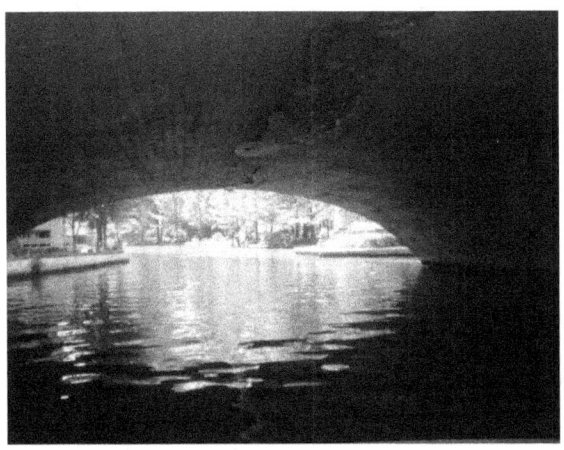

Questions for your consideration:

- Are you comfortable sharing your decisions and journey through infertility with family and friends? Is this what is best for you and your partner?

- Have you discussed the boundaries or limits of shared information with family and friends? (How much do they need to know?) Can you identify the *Pros* and *Cons* associated with sharing this information?

  _____
  _____
  _____
  _____
  _____
  _____
  _____
  _____
  _____

How you and your partner address people on the outside should be common ground. This is one point in the journey that you will need to truly hear what each other is trying to communicate. This is a discussion that may not occur one or two times, rather it may be an ongoing conversation between partners. This is essential because during the treatment process, feelings may unexpectedly change.

Can you identify the *Pros* and *Cons* associated with sharing this information? It is imperative that as a team you decide who to discuss this struggle with and how much to share. It can seem like an invasion if both partners are not united with respect to the information that is shared.

_____

_____

_____

_____

_____

_____

_____

_____

_____

_____

_____

_____

_____

_____

_____

_____

This is a very important discussion to have with your partner since positive reinforcement can have a direct effect on positive outcome of the treatment process.

Many issues are involved with the fertility treatment, but the important issues to you and your partner need to be realized, discussed and understood in order for the two of you to travel this road in harmony.

Discuss the outside groups of people surrounding you and your partner. How do you both react to each group? What are your boundaries, how much do you share and are you united in this approach?

_____

_____

_____

_____

_____

_____

_____

_____

_____

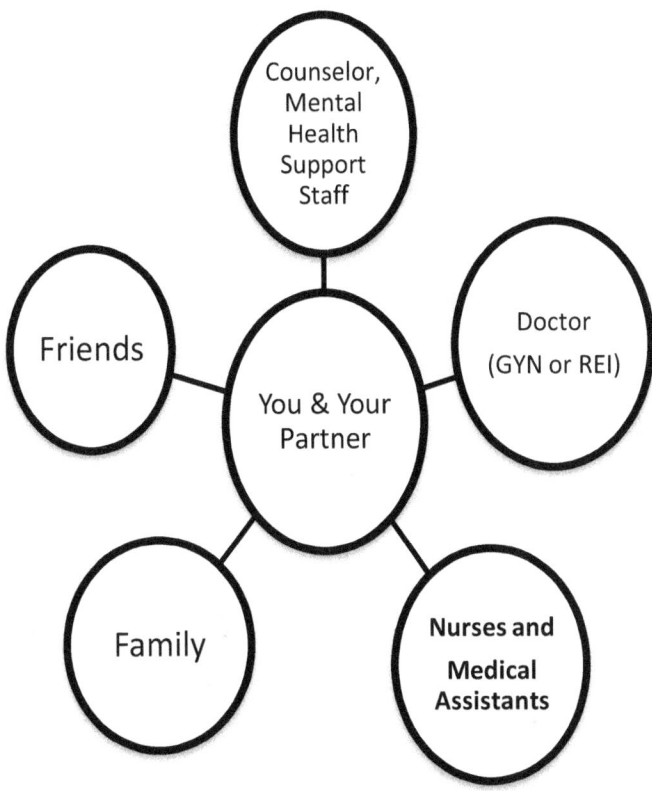

Heart Tip: Know the players on the outside and agree how to handle them as a couple. Identify their "agenda".

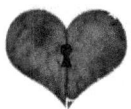

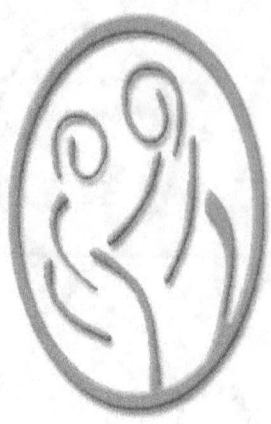

Get the Point?

If you have taken the next treatment step and are taking any medications to regulate your cycle or stimulate follicle growth, please remember that medications can impact your mood!

Lions, Tigers and Bears…Pills, Creams and Injections'….Oh My! We'll get right to the *point* in this section. .. (Sorry, I just couldn't resist the temptation of a good pun).

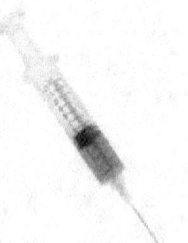

Let's be honest, nobody likes shots and especially more than one shot per day for weeks is not a pleasant thought or experience, but unfortunately often a necessary part of aggressive fertility treatment and certainly the IVF experience.

The positive side of this part of the IVF process is that in most programs your partner is trained to give the necessary injections, allowing you the freedom to carry on with your daily routine with as little disruption as possible.

One couple related the following story about the first time they needed to use injections with a treatment regime. The husband gathered all of the materials necessary for the procedure including the cotton and rubbing alcohol. He very carefully prepared the injection with special attention to measuring the dosage and flicking the tube so as to eliminate air bubbles. The wife noticed a small shot glass filled to the rim with a clear colorless liquid sitting next to the syringe. This peaked her curiosity so she glanced around the room and noted a vodka bottle. With great surprise and a grin she kissed her husband and said "Oh sweetheart, I'm not that nervous… plus I should not drink while we are trying to get pregnant." Her husband looked sheepish, grabbed the shot, smiled and gulped it down saying "OK baby turn around, give me that cute little bottom and let's get this done!" At that moment, she ran out of the room yelling "Oh, I don't think so...."

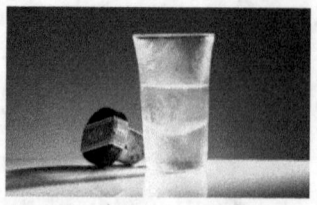

The medications can contribute to the overall anxiety of the process. They can and often do contribute to the emotional experience because they are affecting hormone levels. As your physician controls your cycle, either by suppression or stimulation, you may experience emotional swings. Being aware of the additive effect of the medications to your emotional response is vital to measuring your well being. It is also important for your partner to understand the medications potential impact on your mood swings and reactions.

Heart Tip: Emotional responses should never be discounted as being caused by medications, rather have an understanding that such chemical changes can enhance emotional responses.

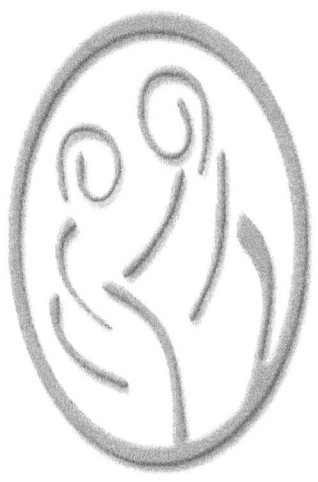

What You <u>Can</u> Do.

According to Dr. Alice Domar at The Mind Body Institute, Harvard Medical School, research shows that patients who increase their ability to adaptively cope with the stressors associated with fertility indicate lower levels of depression. Between identifying the problem, dealing with well meaning family and friends, and trying to solve the problem, you begin to understand the magnitude of emotions that you will be and have been dealing with. I highly recommend any of Dr. Domar's books. Her holistic approach to gaining control of your mind to assist your body is highly insightful and poignant.

There are things that you can do right now to help you through this time in your life. Let's learn some stress and anxiety reducers....

Control what you can...

List three things that you have done for yourself in the last week.

_____

_____

_____

_____

_____

_____

_____

Is that list hard to create or is it expansive? I would be willing to wager that your list of self support and nurturance is ***not*** nearly as long as it should be. Try to make the list again, and write down the ideal list for what you would like to do for yourself in the coming week. Can you create the ideal plan?

_____

_____

_____

_____

_____

_____

_____

_____

_____

_____

_____

_____

_____

_____

_____

_____

_____

1. Make a Nutrition Plan – A healthy diet will help promote overall physical and mental well being. Nutrition is imperative when dealing with the challenges of fertility.
2. Visual Imagery – Get your hand on some relaxation CDs or simply close your eyes and visualize a serene environment (that image is completely up to you and your idea of serenity)
3. Exercise (pick one physical activity and do it every day, if even for only 10 minutes)
4. Creating a Relaxation Response.

Progressive Muscle Relaxation -
Learn how to do self directed
progressive muscle relaxation. Close
your eyes and sit or lay down in a
comfortable position. Start at your
feet and tense your toes, holding the
tension for 5 seconds. Then relax the
muscles. Move up your whole body
making various muscle group first
tense and then relax them.
Concentrate on your body and the
feeling of tightening and relaxing.
Remember to continue to breathe
while doing this exercise.

a. *Deep Breathing* – Breathe
from your diaphragm. This
deep breathing is a very
helpful relaxation technique.

b. *Mindfulness* – Take time to
ultra-focus on a normal task.
For example, eat a piece of
chocolate, being completely
aware and mindful of every
detail of that experience. Use
all of your senses to
completely experience the
eating of the candy. Become
mindful of all sensations and
thoughts. Mindfulness allows
us to experience an event in a

deeper more aware manner; it often brings more enjoyment to a regular task.

Explore acupuncture and therapeutic message as means to relax and focus on well being.

Experiment with different stress reduction techniques finding the ones you enjoy and truly gain benefit from implementing. Once you acknowledge that there is a substantial relationship between what your mind perceives and how your body reacts, you are empowered.

Heart Tip; Experience, dabble and play with music, art, physical activity, meditation, swimming, writing, reading, deep breathing.... Connect your body and mind.

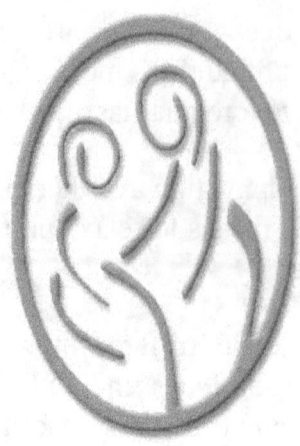

If You Are Considering IVF, You Must Discuss....

In Vitro Fertilization (IVF) is an invasive medical procedure that you may choose to attempt to create your family. The medical professionals who may be treating you will explain IVF from a medical perspective. This procedure involves stimulating the female partner to create follicles containing eggs. These are retrieved from the women in a surgical procedure under conscious sedation. The retrieved eggs are combined with sperm from the male partner and with luck, fertilization will occur. If and when the eggs fertilize, embryos may develop.

The specifics of how many embryos are created and to what stage of development they grow before transfer is scheduled, has numerous interactive influencing elements. IVF is a highly scientific procedure that often results in creating a new life and helping to create and build a family.

IVF is an invasive procedure that promotes intense emotional responses; and that is before the effect of the stimulation medications. The decision to try IVF and the treatment regime is a pivotal time in your relationship, as you may feel optimistic, fearful and extremely vulnerable, simultaneously. The basic stages of IVF are: Cycle Suppression, Stimulation, Monitoring, Egg Retrieval, Fertilization, Transfer of Embryos and the Pregnancy Wait. For our purposes here, I will not describe each of these stages, that is better explained by a medical professional. Each phase of this procedure holds unique emotional aspects and challenges. I have found that the most challenging phase for couples is the transfer procedure and the agonizing long wait for treatment results.

The transfer of the fertilized embryo(s) back into the uterus where the embryo should implant and grow is often overwhelming. It is this moment that you realize you have some level of life growing inside you... You just hope and pray that it will remain, attach and grow.

The transfer stage is a major milestone in the IVF program because it means that you have had some success with fertilization of the eggs. Again, it is important to understand what the procedure of transfer entails and how it will be done, to reduce the level of anxiety and fear of the unknown. This should be discussed with your physician and your IVF nurse prior to your scheduled date of transfer.

For someone challenged by infertility, the following questions are essential and must be considered, even though it may feel unjust or surreal to you.

If more than one egg is fertilized and viable, have you discussed with your partner and your physician how many eggs should be transferred? Consider quality versus quantity issues.

_____
_____
_____
_____
_____
_____
_____
_____

Have you discussed the ramifications
(i.e. physical, emotional and financial)
of multiple successful embryo
implantations?   Consider pregnancy
with twins, triplets or quadruplets….
Remember the goal is one healthy child.

_____
_____
_____
_____
_____
_____
_____

Have you discussed single embryo
transfer?

_____
_____
_____
_____

If more eggs are fertilized than can be used, have you considered and discussed alternative plans for additional fertilized eggs? (i.e. cryopreservation or medical research, disposal, or embryo donation).

_____
_____
_____
_____
_____
_____
_____
_____

Do you believe that your partner has considered any alternative plans for additional fertilized eggs?

_____
_____
_____
_____
_____
_____
_____
_____

Heart Tip: Remember it is out of your
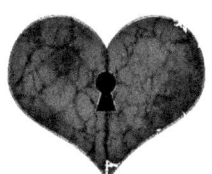 control except for
following medical
instructions.

Regardless of your
religious or spiritual
beliefs; ponder the serenity prayer.

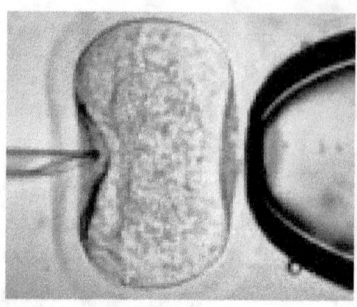

What if it works and what if it doesn't?

Discussion of the treatment outcome is essential. You do not need to have answers to all of the "What if" questions, rather it is helpful to have an idea of your partner's feelings on some of these big questions.

Depending on the number of transferred embryos, multiple embryos may implant. In some cases, selective reduction may be advised by your physician. Selective reduction is the procedure of eliminating one or more implanted embryos for the purpose of ensuring that other embryos will prosper and thrive, as well as for the safety of the mother. Have you considered the possibility of this procedure and how you could feel about it?

a.) Can you identify what issues you would have, if any, with selective reduction?

b.) Do you feel that consulting religious leaders or other professionals, such as mental health counselors, would be of help before having to make this decision?

c.) Can you identify what issues your partner would have, if any, with selective reduction?

d.) When do you believe that life begins and what choices are acceptable to you and your partner?

There are no right choices...

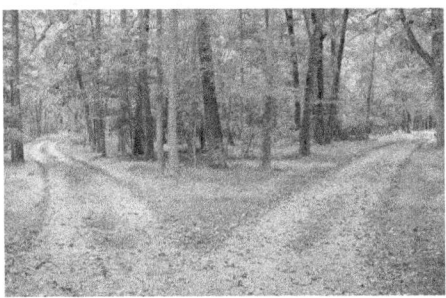

Just better choices for you and your partner.

Being on the same page with these issues is imperative. These are things that must be addressed to some degree before you are in the middle of them...

There can be difficult choices that require your careful thought and attention. Such decisions are best addressed when you have a comfortable and trusting relationship with your physician.

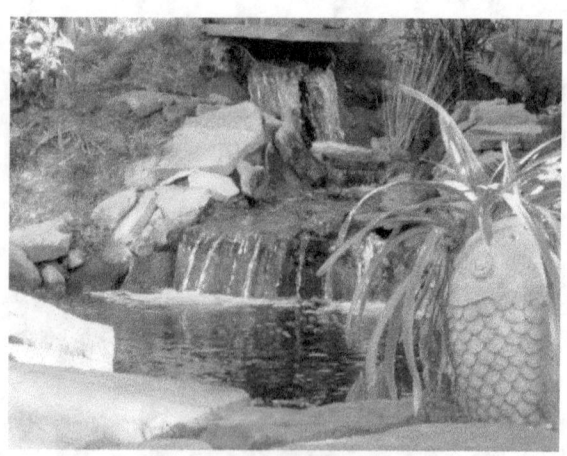

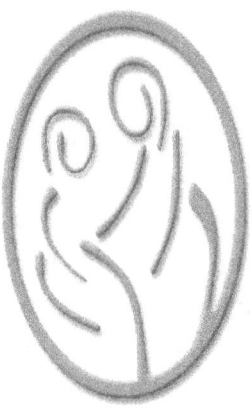

The Longest Wait…
IUI or IVF

Twelve to fourteen days doesn't seem like a very long time, why it's just two weeks, unless of course you are waiting to find out if all you have gone through was worth it. Now you are talking about an eternity, or so it seems.

The first week is the worst; it is like time just came to a halt. Take control and take a trip…. It helps to have a plan.

1. Discuss the possibility of travel with your partner and your physician.

More than likely you are going to be mentally and physically tired at this stage of the program and a relaxing trip somewhere you both enjoy would be beneficial. It has been our experience to recommend a place that is familiar, pleasant and comfortable to you to eliminate any stress of the unknown. Make a list of five places that you would enjoy going to and ask your partner to do the same. Take a quiet evening and discuss your options and choose your destination.

2. If travel is not an option, make a list of activities that you both enjoy doing, and then share your ideas. The most important aspect of the waiting period is to remain busy. For example:

- See a movie. (list a few you have wanted to see… comedies are a great choice now)
- Pick a few new restaurants and then try new foods at each.
- Investigate sporting and/ or cultural events coming in the next two weeks and plan on attending them together.
- Go shopping and buy something unusual that both of you would enjoy.

- Find an exciting new book to read during this period.

The key is to pick activities that you can do together and enjoy each other's company. Supporting each other, discussing your feelings and sharing this time together will give you strength and confidence. If you have a strong support network of friends and family plan some activities and time with them. It is important to seek out positive support from as many aspects of your life as possible during this, what seems to be a forever waiting period.

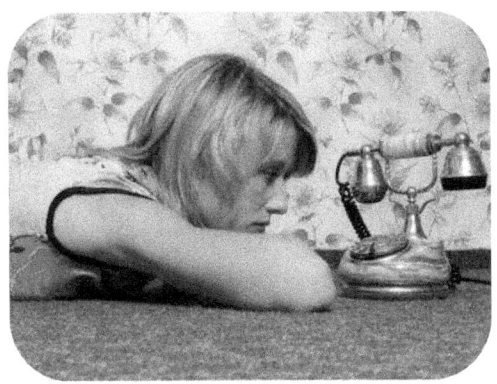

The call will come…

In twelve to fourteen days you will take a blood test and your physician or nurse will call you and let you know if the procedure has been successful or not. You will receive your beta HcG number indicating the presence of a pregnancy.

If the answer is yes, tears of joy and overwhelming relief will pass through you, as you have never felt before. The experience is virtually surreal, and the level of emotion that you will feel is almost indescribable. You will have the feeling that you and your partner have finally become one in heart, body and spirit.

Sometimes, we must be prepared for the answer of maybe. What we mean by maybe is that sometimes the "numbers" (beta HcG) indicate that there is a pregnancy, but perhaps not a healthy pregnancy. This is a very difficult position to be in because you want to be excited with your possible success, but you are afraid of the loss that you might incur.

This unexpected result is extremely challenging because there 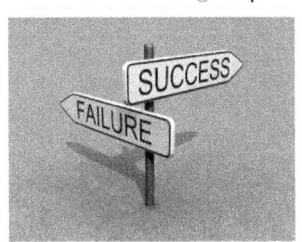 may be no definitive answer for a period of time. You should request a meeting with your physician and ask him or her to please explain what your numbers indicate and how likely your chances are for a successful pregnancy at this point.

It is very important that if at all possible, both partners participate in this meeting with your physician. Unfortunately, not all outcomes are positive. Even as far as medical science has come in this field, nothing is for sure and there are no guarantees. You think you understand all the ramifications in the beginning of your treatment journey, but somehow it doesn't make hearing the answer of no, any easier in the end. Nothing can cushion the depth of the blow that has been handed to you, and it sometimes feels as if you will never recover from the disappointment and the hurt. Some of our patients have even described the feelings as being comparable to experiencing a loss due to death.

The mind, body and spirit have a remarkable ability to withstand much more than we believe we are capable of, and sometimes this is tested to the limit of what we believe we can handle. What you should remember is that there are always alternatives to achieving your goals. Whether you pursue additional medical interventions or explore alternate parenting choices, you can achieve your goal of having a family.

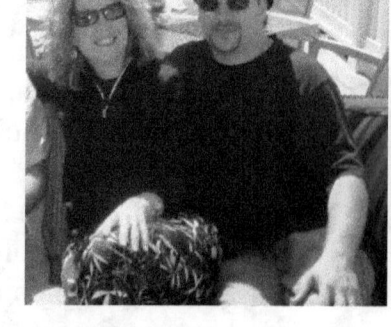

The absolute key to surviving this journey is taking it with your partner. Journey together in your hopes, your fears, your successes and your disappointments….

Heart Tip: This all must be endured hand in hand and back to back. Support one another with unconditional love.

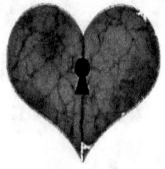

Final Thoughts

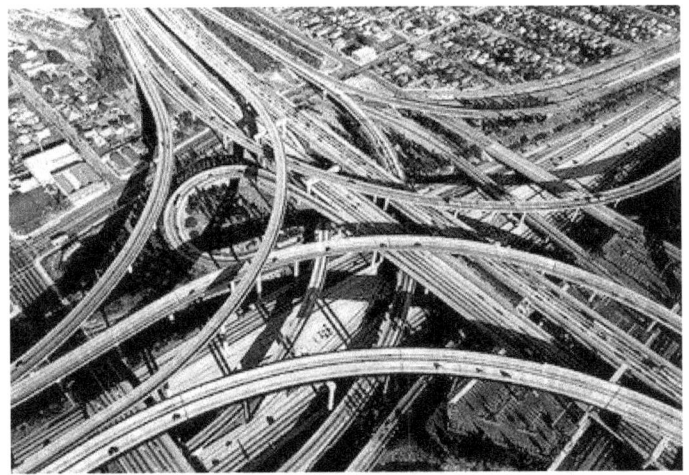

Infertility is no longer *The Road Less Traveled*... today our numbers are growing and our voices are audible.

The diagnosis of infertility is not a choice, rather it is an unexpected life changing road that you were forced to take. However, how well you travel that road is largely up to you.

Reach out and find support services that can provide information about your diagnosis and possible treatment regimes. Find healthy outlets for your anxiety and frustration. Express your feelings and identify your beliefs. Be aware that this time in your life will pass and where you end this journey will have been determined by your perseverance and your motivation. Care for yourself and your partner paying special attention to your psychological needs. In other words... listen to your heart.

Heart Tip: Hold onto one another and be open to the idea that your road may take you places you never imagined, but there are gifts inherent in the journey. Follow the road as far as you can; regrets are not baggage you need. Choose your physician with care and diligence. Consider that changing roads sometimes gets you to your destination via an unplanned route.

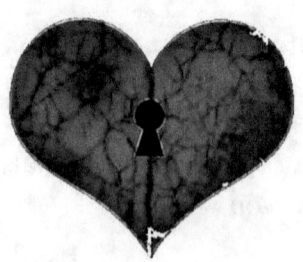

Jim and I learned many of these lessons on our own seven year journey. We endured six IUI attempts, two IVF cycles, and a painful miscarriage of twins. We genuinely found each other on this journey by holding on

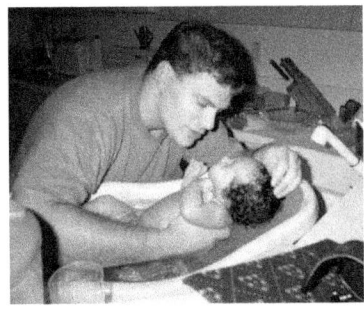

tight and learning how to support the other, unconditionally. To say the least, it was a challenge.

We have no regrets about the choices we made on our journey; in the end, we adopted our beautiful daughter. We found the child we believe we were always meant to have. The promise of parenthood can be within reach if you hold on, fight for each other and fight for the dream.

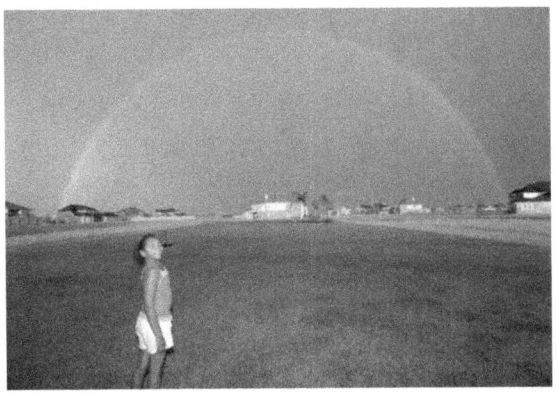

<u>*Acknowledgements*</u>

Special thanks and appreciation to my mom and dad for years of support and their unwavering desire to be Grandparents.

Thank you to my best friend and husband Jim, who took this journey with me, hand in hand.

This book is dedicated to Sydney Gail who was waiting at the end of our rainbow.

To contact Cristina Treadway

<u>InsighTX@gmail.com</u>

<u>www.MyInfertilityResources.com</u>

Cristina is a Texas Licensed Professional Counselor